HEALING STRESS

EFFECTIVE SOLUTIONS FOR RELIEVING STRESS AND LIVING A STRESS-FREE LIFE

THOMAS CALABRIS

Check out our website at:

www.EliminateStressNow.com

Healing Stress

Publisher : Inner Vitality Systems, LLC.
Website : www.EliminateStressNow.com
ISBN : 978-1-7329106-2-1

Copyright © 2018 by Thomas Calabris

Disclaimer

The Information presented in this publication is intended as an educational resource and is not intended as a substitute for proper medical advice. All readers are encouraged to seek proper professional and medical advice when needed. This book is not for anyone that has medical mental conditions. Do not read this book and seek proper medical treatment if you have serious mental illness.

The author and publisher of this material are not responsible in any manner whatsoever for any action or injury which may occur by reading or following the instruction in this document. The author cannot be held responsible for any personal or commercial damage caused by misinterpretation of the information or improper use of the information.

No patent liability is assumed with respect to the use of the information contained herein. Although every precaution

Healing Stress

has been taken in the preparation of this book, the publisher and author assume no responsibility for errors or omissions.

TABLE OF CONTENTS

Healing Stress

CHAPTER 1 – INTRODUCTION

"The greatest weapon against stress is our ability to choose one thought over another."

- William James

Each day it seams as though there are more and more reasons to be stressed out. We can find stress at work, at home, in the car, at the doctor's office, and some many other places. Stress is at epidemic levels. However, before we can talk about healing stress, we must understand what stress is.

When we talk about stress, we really should talk about the "stress response". The "stress response" is an evolved survival mechanism in our autonomic nervous system. Our autonomic nervous system receives input or information from our senses and our conscious mind and it has to make split-second decisions about whether we are safe or "under threat" from harm.

If the decision is "under threat", the autonomic nervous system activates the "stress response", otherwise known as the "fight or flight" response. This response can happen so quickly, even before you are even consciously aware that there is a threat present. As a result, the body is prepared, through nervous and hormonal mechanisms to deal with a threat, which can be real or imagined.

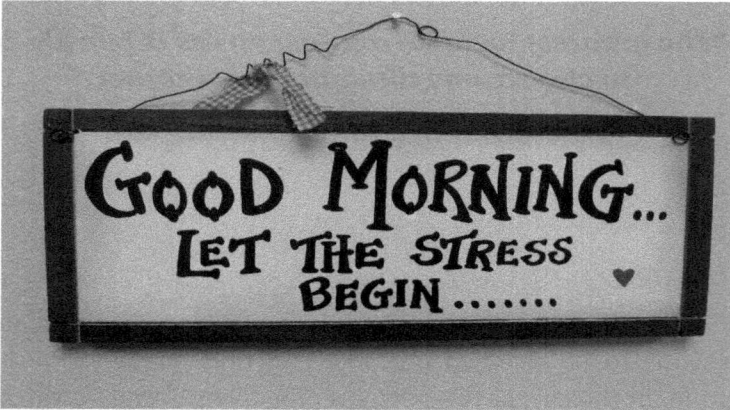

While stress can motivate us to to take action when we face real harm, stress can also cause terrible damage to our overall health if it becomes chronic. That's why it is critical to relieve it immediately.

Life is full of problems, negative people, difficult situations, and unexpected events. Everyone experiences these from time-to-time. But it is the way you perceive and respond to life's challenges that can lead to either great peace or severe stress.

Ultimately it is our choices that determine which one we experience. We can choose an awful life full of stress, tension, grief, and sorrow. Or we can choose an extraordinary life full of happiness, joy, prosperity, and peace.

You know harmful chronic stress is bad for your health. You have heard it over and over from doctors, teachers, friends, and others. So, you know how important it is to get over stress to protect your health and live longer.

In the coming chapters, we will explore what stress is, how it manifests in your mind and body, stress relief options, and how to prevent stress. Of course, we make no claims about being able to completely eliminate stress because it is almost impossible to do.

In some situations, stress is good because it keeps you from harm. It is the chronic stress that occurs because of our mental perception that we must learn to heal and eliminate. We start in the next chapter with what stress is and its effects on the body and the mind.

CHAPTER 2 – STRESS EFFECTS ON THE BODY AND MIND

"Its not stress that kills us, it is our reaction to it."

- Hans Selye

Chronic stress has many negative effects on the body and the mind. However, not all stress is bad. Stress is essential for daily living, and it's only when stress becomes chronic that it can become harmful.

PHYSIOLOGICAL RESPONSE

Physiologically, the stress response signals the adrenal glands to produce the hormones that prepares your body for fight or flight. These hormones include adrenaline, norepinephrine, and cortisol. They are responsible for increasing your heart rate, increasing blood flow to your muscles, and reducing other unnecessary functions until the threat or stressor is past. [1]

4

While stress is known to cause high cortisol levels, chronic stress can lead to adrenal fatigue. When the adrenal glands are fatigued, they produce fewer hormones, which leads to the body's weakened ability to adapt to stress. Low cortisol levels mean that the body is more susceptible to inflammation and fatigue. Blood sugar swings are likely and sodium levels can become depleted, which can lead to dehydration.

While the adrenal glands are more well known to be associated with stress, most people do not know that stress also involves the thymus gland. Stress causes the thymus gland to shrink. And since the thymus gland is part of the immune system, it has an obvious and direct impact on your health. [2]

One typical example of this is when people are under stress, which causes their immune system to be suppressed, and then they end up catching a cold. Long-term stress is harmful because it obstructs the body's natural processes of regeneration and detoxification.

MENTAL AND EMOTIONAL STRESS

In some cases, chronic stress can be attributed to not living in the present moment. It can be attributed to worrying about the future. People worry about many things including getting sick, not having enough money to pay the bills, what other people think about them, whether it will rain, and much more.

Stress can also be caused by being stuck in the past. It is easy to forget all of the good that has happened in our life when there is a lot of negative experiences in our past. People sometimes waste present moments focusing on the negativity from their past. "I remember what so and so did to me. They hurt me." Letting go of the past is important for moving forward and reducing stress.

Worrying can create long-term psychological stress. Even imagined stress can take its toll on the body and the mind. The subconscious mind, which is part of the autonomic nervous system, can't tell the difference between real harm and imagined harm. Both will trigger a stress response.

The stress response will cause your body to suppress growth, repair, healing, digestion, and immune function until the stress has passed. If you live with chronic stress, then the stress response remains turned on and it will cause health issues.

SIGNS OF STRESS

There are numerous signs of stress ranging from mental/emotional to physical symptoms. It is important to recognize that these symptoms overlap with other causes of health issues, so it is important to see your holistic health doctor or practitioner to determine if you have a serious medical condition.

Physical Signs

◆ Rapid heart rate

◆ High blood pressure

◆ Always tired

◆ Fatigue

◆ Weakness

◆ Chest pain

◆ Heart attacks

◆ Insomnia, disturbing dreams, nightmares

◆ Jaw clenching or pain

◆ Stuttering or stammering

◆ Frequent headaches

◆ Sweating

◆ Clammy or cold hands, feet

◆ Difficulty breathing

◆ Frequent urination

◆ Itching

◆ Weight loss or gain without diet changes

Mental/Emotional Signs

◆ Depression

◆ Anxiety

◆ Worry

◆ Suicidal thoughts

◆ Difficulty learning new information

◆ Poor memory

◆ Loss of control

◆ Social withdrawal

◆ Excessive behavior

◆ Mood swings

◆ Guilt

◆ Nervousness

◆ Hostility

These symptoms may be indicative of a serious health or medical condition and if you have any of these you should seek out professional medical attention.

People that live with chronic stress often times look for ways to escape the stress and pain. This escape can take many forms, including using alcohol and drugs to numb the pain (mental or physical). Other forms of escape includes overeating, watching too much TV, and gambling.

Unfortunately, the need to escape stress often times leads to addictions. It is important to know the signs of stress so you can get help before it becomes too much and you need to escape.

CHAPTER 3 – STRESS STUDIES

"It's a good idea always to do something relaxing prior to making an important decision in your life."

- Paulo Coelho

There have been many studies and much research about stress. The studies covered in this chapter will give you a bigger picture about stress.

AMERICANS AND STRESS

The American Psychological Association released a study in 2005 that found a link between six leading causes of death and stress. It was also found that two-thirds of the visits to the doctor were related to stress. And, sixty-four percent of Americans were trying to relieve stress on a daily basis. [3]

WORK STRESS

About half of American workers feel their jobs are very stressful. Some studies indicate that stress at work may be as harmful to your health as smoking or not exercising. A few work related stressors include: lack of job security, unreasonable performance demands, night-shift work, spending too much time on the job and not enough with family. [4]

STRESS AND MORTALITY IN OLDER MEN

According to a study that was published in the Journal of Aging Research, there was a direct correlation between stress levels and mortality in aging men. [5] The study focused on three groups, one with low stress, one with moderate stress, and one with high stress. Both moderate stress and high stress groups showed high mortality.

STRESS AND PREGNANCY

A recent study conducted by the Community Child Health Network looked at cortisol levels in relation to pregnancy. The study found that women that had higher than normal cortisol levels, due to chronic stress, were more likely to have babies with low birth weights (less than about five and a half pounds). Thus, women should consider their stress levels when deciding to get pregnant. [6]

SLEEP LOSS AND STRESS

A survey by the American Psychological Association showed that American adults are only getting on average 6.7 hours of sleep each night. This is less than the recommended 7 to 9 hours of sleep per night. The survey also reported that stress caused 43% of adults to stay awake at night in the past month. Even worse is that 21% felt more stress when they didn't get enough sleep. [7]

SOCIAL MEDIA AND STRESS

According to a Pew Research Center survey, in general, regular users of the internet and social media do not have higher levels of stress. However, there is a link with stress when the social use of digital technology increases the users' awareness of stressful circumstances in the lives of others. Thus, showing the "cost of caring". In general, women reported having more stress than men. [8]

CHAPTER 4 – STRESSORS

"Rule number one is, don't sweat the small stuff.
Rule number two is, it's all small stuff."

- Robert Eliot

Stressors are those situations and events that trigger a stress response. Stressors can be real events and they can be imagined events. For example, an encounter with a wild bear will trigger a stress response because our very survival is at stake. Worrying about taking a test can also cause a stress response. Other stressors include, but are not limited to, health issues, major life events, work, problem relationships, and money.

HEALTH ISSUES

Health issues can weigh on your mind and even become a source of stress. What's worse is that the stress that you feel about your health condition can actually make the condition worse. It can become a vicious cycle if you don't take control of it. Chronic health issues indicate that some aspect of your life is out of balance. Thus, finding a solution to your health issue can also remove a trigger of stress in your life. So, it is important that if your health issues are taking over your life, that you get professional health care from a licensed health care practitioner.

Health issues can also be a source of stress for the loved ones of the person with the issues. They worry about the person and wish for them to get well, but if they let their minds wander into negative territory, they may find themselves feeling stress.

MAJOR LIFE EVENTS

When we think of events like going to college, getting married, or having a baby, we tend to think of the positive aspects and benefits of the events. However, for the person that is anticipating and will partake in the life event, it can become a source of stress. This typically happens when they start to doubt themselves and wonder if they are capable, ready, or worthy of having success at all. That is why it is so important to be positive and stay in the present moment. Avoid going down the path of future *"What Ifs"*. *"What if this doesn't work?"* or *"What if that happens?"* These are things that have yet to happen and are likely not to happen, so let them go.

STRESS AT WORK

We depend on work to provide a source of income so that we can put a roof over our heads, buy food, and provide for our families. So we feel the need and sometimes pressure to work hard to keep the job. So, what happens when you have a difficult work situation or environment? You feel stressed by it, especially if you feel it is out of your control. You don't want to quit, because you are not sure if you can find another job that pays as well.

If you live with this stress day in and day out, then it can take its toll on your health. So, it is best to find a way to turn the situation around. Maybe, you can talk the situation over with your boss. If your boss is the source of the stress, then maybe you can find another position within your company. The bottom line is that you shouldn't just give up and stay with your current job if you are stressed all the time. Keep searching for a solution. It will be better for you and your family in the long run.

STRESS IN RELATIONSHIP

Struggles in relationships can be a big source of stress. This includes everything from disagreements, verbal abuse, and physical abuse. It is important to understand that any abuse should not be tolerated. Other types of disagreements should be approached with loving kindness and compassion. Don't try to ignore the situation, since a lack of communication will only serve to make the situation worse.

If you are in a difficult relationship or even a friendship, it is important to see the other person's point of view even if you don't agree with it. Let go of petty behavior like name calling, accusations, and even lying. In the words of Dr. Wayne Dyer, "It is better to be kind, than right." To what end will it be, if you win the argument and lose a friendship or a spouse? Loving kindness, compassion, and forgiveness should be the cornerstone of every relationship. If you keep this in mind, your relationships will be healthy and less stressful.

STRESS AND MONEY

Money is sometimes called *"The root of all evil."* However, money or the lack thereof, is a huge source of stress for those that struggle to make enough money to pay the bills. Some people have to choose between eating and putting a roof over their families' heads. That is real stress. Imagine not being able to buy your kids the toys they want. Imagine not being able to buy presents for the family at Christmas time. The stress that the lack of money can cause comes in many forms.

Studies show that money is a major cause of stress in relationships. If money is a huge source of your stress, then it is important that you face it with positivity and realism. Being positive can help to soften the stress. And it will help you from attracting more negativity into your life. Being positive is also important for being realistic about solving the issues you face. While it may be realistic to get a better job, it may not be realistic to expect that you will get out of debt in a couple of months. While everyone's situation is different, it is important to learn from your own situation and make a plan to work towards a resolution. Financial counseling may be necessary to get you back on track. Stay positive and never give up.

CHAPTER 5 – STRESS MANAGEMENT

"Doing something that is productive is a great way to alleviate emotional stress. Get your mind doing something that is productive."

- Ziggy Marley

Most people suffer from some form of stress in their everyday lives. Sometimes, they believe that they will not be able to relieve their stress without removing everything in their lives that causes tension. This is usually impossible. However, stress is not something that anyone needs to tolerate, regardless of their situation. There are healthy ways that anyone can do to better handle and relieve the stress in their lives.

You can effectively manage your stress if you know what works and what doesn't work. For example, studies have shown that activities like watching TV, drinking, and smoking reduce mental sharpness and increase the effects of stress. Therefore, watching TV and having drinks are not effective solutions for reducing stress. Yet many people turn to these activities and end up in a worse state since the effects of stress accumulates over time.

The good news is that there are simple and effective ways for managing stress and achieving stress relief. We'll go over some ways here, but these are by no means an exhaustive list. I recommend keeping an open mind and being creative where stress relief is concerned.

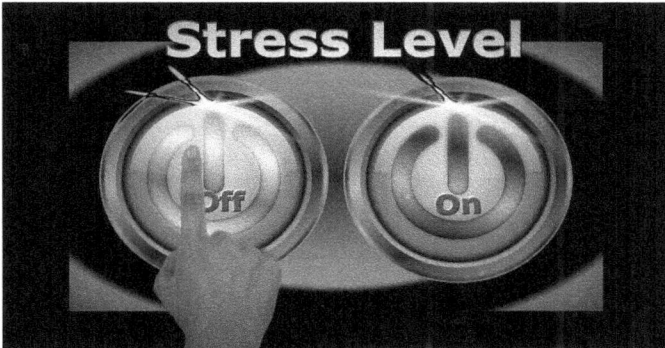

Stress management requires a holistic approach to be effective. It requires mental, emotional, and physical adjustments to make a lasting difference to relieve or eliminate stress. It is the choices that we make that will determine the effectiveness of our stress management strategy.

MENTAL AND EMOTIONAL ADJUSTMENTS

The stress that we experience is often-times caused by a perception that we will be harmed, whether it is true or not. It is our thoughts that are the key to dealing with stress. Therefore, it is important that our thoughts remain rooted in the facts, rather than letting our worries take over our thoughts.

It is important to point out that the root cause of all stress is fear. Fear is a necessary emotion that is essential for self preservation during real life threatening events like natural disasters, house fires, car accidents, and being chased by an angry bear, to name a few. However, when we focus our attention on negative things that could happen to us in the future, we stop living in the present and become afraid of the future.

Thus, the first step to controlling our thoughts and emotions to prevent unnecessary stress caused by unfounded fears, is to focus our attention in the present moment. All we really have is the present moment.

Also, the past is over. Learn from the past and let it go. Often-times we hold onto negative thoughts of the past when we feel as though someone has mistreated us. Living with a grudge and anger keeps us from fully living in the present moment. That's not to say that you should condone the actions of someone that has abused you. But if you hold onto resentment and anger, then you aren't moving forward and you are stuck in the past. Forgive and let go are the keys that will set you free from the past.

By the same token, the future hasn't happened so why waste our present moments worrying about something that may never happen? Everyone has done this a few times or more in their life. *"What if I lose my job?"* or *"What if I never get a job?"* or *"What if he doesn't like me?"* or *"What if I flunk the test?"*. This kind of worrying is not productive and it causes us to attract the very things that we are worrying about. Like attracts like.

So, changing your perception of an upcoming event and seeing it as an adventure or a positive challenge can alleviate the stress. Avoid amplifying the issues of an event. Don't repeat the possible negative aspects of the event over and over in your mind. Do not see it as a *"punishment"*. Avoid over dramatizing it. Maintain objectivity as much as possible. Don't take things personally.

When we consistently worry about the future, we are training our subconscious mind to fear future events. This is how we become afraid of change itself. Our subconscious mind is programmed by the daily thoughts that we have. When the daily thoughts are negative and have a fear-based tone, we set ourselves up for living with stress on a regular basis.

It is very important that we learn to identify the fears that are causing our stress, so we can learn to deal with and eliminate them. Whenever you find yourself in a stressful situation, ask yourself (without judgments), *"What is the fear that is causing me to have a stress response?"* Look deeply inside at what you are thinking and feeling. I recommend writing down your stressors and your fears in a journal so that you can reflect on them and find solutions to eliminate and prevent them.

PHYSICAL ADJUSTMENTS

It is often the case that we can better handle stress if we make physical adjustments in our lives. While the cause of our stress may be mental or emotional, we can reduce the effects of stress if we make some adjustments to our lifestyle. This includes eating healthier, getting plenty of sleep, exercising, and laughing more. We will go over some of these in greater details in future chapters.

PRACTICE ACCEPTANCE

People often feel stress when they feel that they cannot control some circumstance in their lives. One way to handle this is to recognize what you can control and what you can't control. It is best to learn to accept the things you cannot control. For instance, if you are stuck in a traffic jam and find yourself becoming upset over being late to a meeting or a social event, you can say to yourself: *"I have no control over this situation. I will get there when I get there."* This takes away the additional pressure that comes with being upset or being nervous about the situation.

WRITE IT DOWN

One major symptom of stress is that people lose a lot of sleep because they are awake all night worrying about their problems. One way to handle this is by writing down the problems and potential solutions before bed. This way you can rest easy knowing that you have a plan for the next day.

KICK THE HABIT

Many people take up the unhealthy habit of smoking because they believe that it reduces their stress. Medically, this is simply not true because nicotine, which is a stimulant, actually increases stress symptoms. Quitting smoking will eliminate the stimulant induced stress symptoms, and will eliminate the potential bad health consequences of smoking in the future.

TAKE A HOT SHOWER OR BATH

It is beneficial to take a hot shower or bath when you feel stressed. The hot water helps to relax your muscles. You can add Epsom Salts to your bath for additional relief. The Epsom Salts contains magnesium, which helps muscles to relax.

GET A MASSAGE

Get a massage from a licensed massage therapist. A massage will help to release the tension in your body that was caused by stress. Types of massage to consider are deep tissue, Swedish massage, Shiatsu, reflexology, acupressure, and Tai massage.

GET AN ACUPUNCTURE TREATMENT

This is a method from Traditional Chinese Medicine (TCM) that involves inserting very thin needles into points, called acupuncture points, in the body to balance the natural flow of energy through your body. Since stress can cause blockages in the flow of energy in the body, acupuncture is a good way to release the blockages. If you don't like needles, then you can try acupressure, which releases the energy blockages by massaging the acupuncture points.

RELAXATION TECHNIQUE

A great way to release stress is to practice the progressive relaxation technique. Lie down in a comfortable position with your legs uncrossed and your arms at your sides. Start at your feet. Consciously tense the muscles of your feet and allow them to relax. Do this for each muscle group from your feet to your head and then repeat them again. This will leave you feeling more relaxed and rejuvenated.

HYPNOTHERAPY

Hypnotherapy is a technique where a hypnotherapist puts their client under a hypnotic state and gives them suggestions to modify their behavior, such as to relax and to let go of what is stressing them. There are some techniques that allow for self-hypnosis between sessions.

TURN OFF ELECTRONICS

Turn off your electronic devices. Constantly checking emails and social media posts can be consuming. These days most people are constantly seeking a connection with someone online. Cell phones give us instant non-verbal communications through text messaging. People feel obligated to respond immediately to requests to chat, emails, and posts.

It's beneficial to take an electronic break. Believe it or not, you are not obligated to respond immediately to every inquiry. Here's one for you. You don't have to answer your cell phone while you are on the toilet. Have you ever been talking to someone on the cell phone and heard the toilet flush in the background? Hang up and do your business. The world won't end if you take a break. There's nothing wrong with using electronic devices, but you must use them in moderation, otherwise you run the risk of becoming addicted to them. Then, it will take over and rule your life.

LAUGHTER

Laughter is a great way to relieve the effects of stress. Studies have shown that laughter can not only relieve stress, but it can also boost your immune function, and relieve pain. Laughing induces a relaxation response in the body. As a result, laughing reduces the production of stress hormones. It also increases the feel good neurotransmitters in the brain, like endorphins and serotonin, thus improving our mood. [9]

There are so many ways to get your dose of laughter these days. Options range from watching a situation comedy on TV, watching a funny movie, watching funny video clips on the internet, and more. Most options are inexpensive. Laughter is even better when you share something funny with your family and friends.

This chapter gave you a bird's eye view of stress management ideas and techniques to get you started. The remaining chapters are dedicated to either stress relief or stress prevention.

CHAPTER 6 – POSITIVE SELF-IMAGE

"What lies behind us and what lies before us are tiny matters compared to what lies within us."

- Ralph Waldo Emerson

Having a positive self-image is important for leading a happy, healthy, and stress-free life. How you see yourself determines your self-worth. How do you see yourself? Do you feel good about who you are and what you do on a daily basis? Write these questions and your answers in your journal. Reflect on these questions daily. If you are truly working towards a stress-free life, you will see that your answers to these questions will be different from the first time you answered them. This is a sign of progress.

YOU ARE WORTHY

It is important to recognize that just based on the fact that you were born into this world, you are worthy of all of the abundance in the universe. You are as worthy of love and

27

happiness as much as anyone on the planet now or that has ever lived.

Sometimes during our childhood, we have been told so many times that we weren't good enough. That we shouldn't get our hopes up. That we shouldn't expect too much out of life. You can't do this or that. Sometimes this negativity comes from bullies. Sometimes this negativity comes from people we care about.

If this kind of negativity has been ingrained into your psyche, you may feel unworthy. Fortunately, they were wrong and you are worthy. The next time you see yourself in the mirror, say to yourself, *"I love you and I am worthy of all of the abundance in the universe."* Repeat this to yourself every morning. Eventually, you will begin to feel it and even believe it.

CHANGE YOUR SELF-TALK

One way to reduce the amount of stress in your life is to change your self-talk. Most often our self-talk or inner dialogue is negative. This negative self-talk not only increases stress, but it limits our self-worth and our self-image. Thus, it is time to change the tone of our self-talk to one that is positive and empowering. It is our inner thoughts that help us to manifest the world we live in.

This inner dialogue sends out an energy with an energetic frequency. And, we attract people, things, and circumstances that match the energy frequencies that we send out. This is known as the *"Law of Attraction"*.

The type and tone of our self-talk will program our subconscious mind over time. Then, at some point, we will have this internal dialog, but we won't be conscious about it. It becomes unconscious thoughts. Let me rephrase this so you understand. It is the thoughts, positive or negative, that we repeat on a regular basis, that programs our subconscious mind.

For example, let's say you grew up in a not so loving home, where you were constantly belittled and criticized. And you were constantly having to defend yourself. You may have felt that people treated you unfairly. At some point, all of these negative thoughts become unconscious if we allow it to continue for very long. Then one day, the negative thoughts start, but in an unconscious way. And they may be directed at yourself instead of others. They may also become reactionary, let's say, when someone criticizes you, you may react with anger instead of realizing that they were giving you good advice.

So, you may be wondering, what do we do to eliminate these unconscious negatively programmed thoughts? In theory it is simple. Just make a choice to think positive, empowering, loving, and compassionate thoughts. It is our conscious choices of the thoughts that we think that ultimately program our subconscious mind. By making our conscious thoughts positive, we will change the unconscious programming over time. We must be patient when we are retraining our subconscious mind.

Now as we are reprogramming our subconscious mind, an interesting thing happens, we also change our physiology. We will stop feeding the stress response, which is governed by the sympathetic nervous system, and we begin to activate the relaxation response, which is governed by the parasympathetic nervous system.

When the parasympathetic nervous system is most dominant, the physiology of relaxation, healing, repair, and detoxification can happen naturally. Our immune system is no longer suppressed and it gets stronger. The tension in our muscles release and we become more relaxed than we thought was possible. Our mind also relaxes and the positive thoughts or self-talk attract positive and beneficial things into our lives.

POSITIVE AFFIRMATIONS

Positive affirmations are a great way for you to retrain your mind to have a positive inner dialogue. Repeat as many positive affirmations as you can when you wake up and before you go to sleep at night. One of my favorite positive affirmations is *"I am calm, peaceful, and relaxed in this moment."* Other positive affirmations include, *"I am courageous."* or *"I am peaceful and joyful."* Now it is your turn to take action and create a positive affirmation that represents the positive outcome you would like to achieve. Be creative and as always, have fun with it.

VISUALIZATION

Another powerful way to retrain your subconscious mind is through visualization. By visualizing what we want, we can imprint positive and empowering images into our subconscious mind. The subconscious mind doesn't know the difference between that which is imagined and that which is real. To be most effective, our visualizations should use as many of the five senses as possible. "What does it look like?" "How does it feel?" "What does is smell like?" You get the idea. Be as detailed as possible. Use your imagination and be creative.

For example, if you want to learn how to relax, then visualize what your perfect relaxed situation looks like. Perhaps you feel very relaxed when walking in the park. So, imagine walking down the path, surrounded by lots of trees. Feel the warm wind on your face. Hear the sounds of the birds chirping in the background. See the ducks swimming in the pond. You feel so peaceful. You take a deep breath and let it out slowly. You say to yourself, "I feel so calm, peaceful, and relaxed." Be creative. Repeat your visualization every day. Make it fun and enjoyable. I recommend writing down your visualization in words to help you remember it so you can practice it daily.

You will notice that over time, you will begin to create and attract into your life those things that you visualize on a daily basis. Don't take my word for it. Try it for yourself.

CHAPTER 7 – MINDFULNESS PRACTICES

"It's a good idea to always do something relaxing prior to making an important decision in your life."

- Paulo Coelho

The term mindfulness refers to being fully conscious in the present moment. This can have different meanings depending upon your intention in the moment. It can refer to being aware of what is going on in your mind and your body. While it is about awareness, it isn't about being judgmental. It means that you witness what is going on without judgments.

It can also mean being fully aware of what is going on in your environment. For example, if you are walking in nature, like at the park, then you are mindful when you are in the present moment appreciating the nature that is around you. You are not thinking about what happened yesterday or what may happen later. It is about being present in the now, or as I like to call it, the "here and now".

There are many types of mindfulness practices. These include, but are not limited to, meditation, breathing, Yoga, Tai Chi, Qigong, and simply walking. Just about anything can become a mindfulness practice if done with the intention and awareness in the present moment.

For example, washing the dishes can be a mindfulness practice. So, when you are washing the dishes, just wash the dishes. Don't think about anything other than the soap, water, and cleaning the dishes. Be present with the feeling of the warm water, the smell of the soap, and the sound of the running water.

In the following sections, I will go over some mindfulness practices the can help to center you in the present moment and will benefit your health and well-being. See if one of these practices resonates with you and try it out.

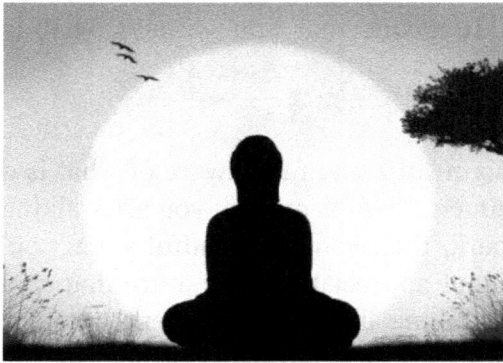

MEDITATION

Meditation is a general term that means to turn your attention inward to your mind and body. There are many different forms of meditation. There are meditations to focus the mind, to calm the mind, to relax the body, to heal the body, to retrain the mind, to enhance the energy flow in the body, to release negative emotions, and many more. It is important to be in the present moment when meditating. A very simple but effective meditation for focusing the mind is to repeat a mantra or an affirmation for a few minutes or more. Meditation induces a relaxation response. Thus, it is important to meditate daily to reduce the effects of stress.

BREATHING

Breathing is a basic function of life and because it comes with an autopilot, the autonomic nervous system of the brain, we often take it for granted. However, we can control our breathing with our conscious mind. Being mindful of your breathing is a great way to relax and energize your mind and body. First, when I refer to breathing for the purpose of this discussion, I am referring to abdominal breathing, which is sometimes referred to as belly breathing. Abdominal breathing means as you inhale deeply, you allow your abdomen to expand. Then as you exhale, you retract your abdomen. You can count your breaths to help focus your mind. At first, it requires extra concentration until you get used to doing it. This requires daily practice. Practice abdominal breathing for a few minutes or longer while you are stressed to help you calm down. You can also benefit by practicing when you aren't stressed as well.

TAI CHI

Tai Chi is a soft style form of martial arts. It is sometimes described as meditation in motion. It is a slow motion form of martial arts movements that enhance the flow of energy in the body. There are many different forms of Tai Chi. It is important to be in the present moment while focusing on each movement. Tai Chi requires proper form, posture, abdominal breathing, and mind focus. Consistent practice of Tai Chi will not only quiet your mind, but it will build strength and energy in your body.

QIGONG

Qigong is a combination of exercises, breathing, and meditation originally developed in China over thousands of years. There are many different forms of Qigong. The foundation of most forms of Qigong is to open the energy channels in the body, build more energy in the body, and to enhance the energy flow. Qigong is practiced for self-healing, health, wellness, illness prevention, healing of others, longevity, and spirituality. The practice of Qigong requires being in the present moment. Consistent practice of Qigong will develop a calm and focused mind.

YOGA

Yoga is most popularly known for the physical aspect of holding specific poses and stretching. Yoga originated in India and there are many different forms of Yoga, including physical poses, mindfulness, meditation, and spiritual practices. Yoga will develop a strong body and a calm and relaxed mind with consistent practice. Yoga is practiced for improving one's health and wellness, peace of mind, and for spiritual purposes.

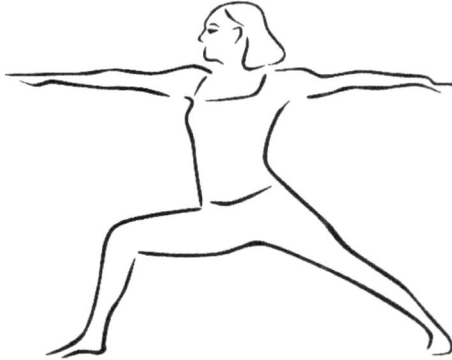

WALKING

Walking while keeping one's awareness in the present moment is another form of mindfulness. Walking in nature is a great way to appreciate the beauty of nature and calm the mind. I recommend doing abdominal breathing while walking where ever you walk. Walking is a good way to get some exercise and if done mindfully, it can focus and calm your mind.

Now it is up to you to make a choice and incorporate a mindfulness practice into your daily life. It is best to choose a practice that resonates with you. There are no right or wrong answers. Just go with your intuition and what feels right for you. I recommend these mindfulness practices as an addition to the other techniques presented in this book.

CHAPTER 8 – SLEEP FOR STRESS RELIEF

"Stress is when you wake up screaming and you realize you haven't fallen asleep yet."

- Author Unknown

Getting the proper amount of sleep is very important for managing or preventing stress. According to the Natural Sleep Foundation, adults need seven to ten hours of sleep each night. Children require more. [10]

During sleep, the body heals and rebuilds. It is also the time when the brain converts short-term memory into long-term memory. If you lose too much sleep, for too many consecutive days, you accumulate sleep debt.

INSOMNIA

Insomnia is a disorder where you have either difficulty falling asleep or staying asleep. It is estimated that between 50 and 70 million U.S. adults have some form of sleep issues. [11] According to the CDC, a survey found that about four percent of US adults age twenty and older used prescription sleeping aids in the previous month. [12]

For someone that lives with chronic stress, they may have problems sleeping because of a racing mind, anxiety, depression, inflammation or pain in the body, or possibly because of some other health condition. Insomnia can also be a side effect of some medications.

Chronic insomnia can cause a wide array of symptoms including:

◆ Low energy

◆ Poor concentration

◆ Fatigue

◆ Irritability

◆ Worsened stress symptoms

◆ Weakened immune function

◆ Poor memory

SLEEP LOSS

Sleep loss triggers your body to increase the levels of hormones produced by the adrenal glands. These hormones, called glucocorticoids, are released during a stress response. Glucocorticoid hormones include norepinephrine, adrenaline, and cortisol. They are designed to keep you attentive. Therefore, with high levels of these hormones circulating in your body, they will at a minimum affect the quality of your sleep, if not inhibit your ability to sleep.

Even modest amounts of sleep loss can cause health issues or more. One sleep study found that getting less than 4 hours of sleep per night yielded a 2.8 times higher rate of mortality for men and a 1.5 times higher rate for women. This study also found that the amount of sleep or lack thereof, was a better indicator of mortality than smoking, cardiac disease, or hypertension. [13]

Another study found that getting six hours or less of sleep a night had a seventy percent higher mortality rate over a nine-year period than those who got seven to eight hours of sleep each night. [13]

So, it is important to get an adequate amount of sleep to relieve the effects of stress. And, it's important to avoid having a lack of sleep being the cause of more stress.

REM SLEEP

The type of sleep that we get is as important as the amount of sleep. Sleep is a combination of REM (rapid eye movement) and non-REM sleep. It is during REM sleep that we dream, our eyes move rapidly, our heart rate is increased, and our breathing is more active. It is during the non-REM sleep that our heart rate is slower and our muscles become relaxed. So, if we are stressed out and our sleep is disturbed, as is the case with insomnia, then we are mostly not getting adequate amounts of REM and non-REM sleep. [14]

DISCONNECT

It is a known fact that the light emitted by electronic devices, like cell phones, interferes with the pineal gland's production of melatonin, which is a hormone that regulates our sleep and wake cycles. The light causes a reduced production of melatonin, which can lead to insomnia. Thus, it is best to disconnect the electronic devices about an hour before bed. Keep them out of the bedroom if at all possible.

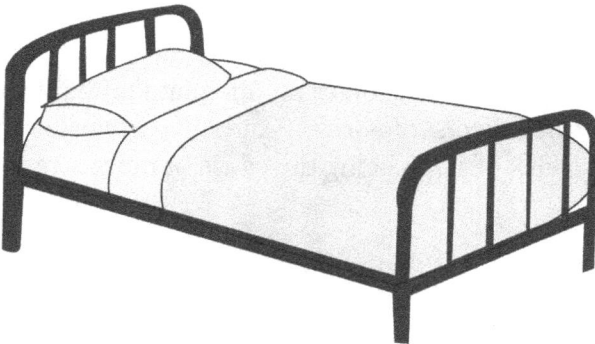

Environment for Sleeping

You can improve your ability to sleep by making some changes to your sleep environment. First, as we have discussed previously, disconnect your electronic devices before bed. Also, for a good night's sleep, it is best to keep the bedroom temperature on the cool side. Of course, it goes without saying, but you need a comfortable mattress to avoid a painful back. Also, lavender essential oil is known for its relaxing qualities. You can put a few drops of lavender on your pillow case to induce relaxation. Avoid waking to the loud sound of an alarm clock. It will startle you and activate a stress response. You can find a CD or an app that has instrumental music that gradually increases the volume over a five-minute period. There are also lights that are programmable to gradually increase in intensity over a short time.

Tips for Getting a Good Night Sleep

1. Go to sleep and wake up at the same time every day.

2. Avoid electronic devices about an hour before bed.

3. Get regular exercise.

4. Avoid stimulants, including caffeine in the afternoon and evening.

5. Calm your mind by focusing on your breathing while in bed.

6. Avoid napping unless it's absolutely necessary.

7. Stop eating food at least several hours before bed.

CHAPTER 9 – EXERCISE FOR STRESS RELIEF

"Turn your face to the sun and the shadows fall behind you."

- Maori Proverb

It is important to consider exercise for improving one's health. Exercises like walking, jogging, Yoga, Tai Chi, Qigong, aerobics, strength training, and more, each have their own benefits for improving one's health.

EXERCISE BENEFITS

Exercise is not only essential for being healthy and staying fit, but it is also beneficial for relieving the effects of stress. Exercise helps by burning off excess stress hormones, thus providing relief from the symptoms caused by stress. It also increases blood flow and therefore oxygen to the brain, thus lessening fatigue.

Increased blood flow to the brain also helps to improve mental clarity, giving way to better problem solving and thereby relieving the mental aspects of stress. Exercise also releases so called "feel good" neurotransmitters called endorphins that can give you the "runner's high" and relieves physical pain. [15] This can also help lessen the feelings of anxiety and depression. And, getting physically fit can also boost your self-esteem because you feel healthy.

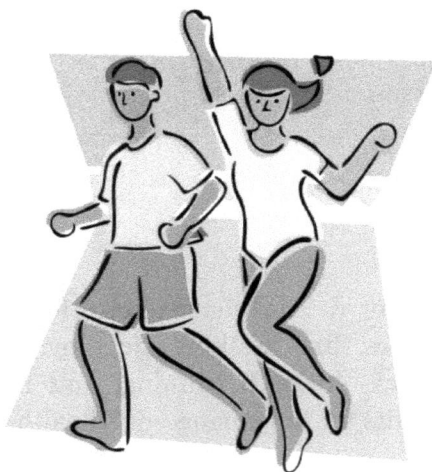

Sweating during physical workouts helps to eliminate toxins in the body through the skin. Exercise also increases the flow of lymph thereby helping to remove toxins.

Other benefits of exercising include decreasing tension, increasing muscle tone, increasing physical endurance, losing weight, enhancing the mind-body connection, improving sleep, and increasing bone density to name a few.

To really get the benefits from exercise you need to be consistent and practice regularly.

WARMING UP

Warming up before exercise can help to prevent injuries. Warming up increases blood circulation and body temperature. This prevents muscle cramps and tearing of muscles, tendons, and ligaments. Start out slow and gradually build up to more moderate activity to avoid injuries. About five minutes is all you really need to properly warm-up. Warming up can include more gentle types of movements, including rotating your arms, legs, wrists, and feet in each direction. You can also move your knees and elbows to warm them up. Make sure you warm-up before stretching as well as other exercises.

DON'T OVER EXERCISE

It is important that you don't over exercise when you are under chronic stress because too much exercise can increase your level of stress hormones. Over time, you could weaken your adrenal glands by exercising too much. If you have adrenal fatigue, too much exercise could further exhaust your adrenal glands and may cause inflammation in the body. That is why for chronic stress and adrenal fatigue, I recommend focusing on lighter types of exercise including mindfulness practices like Yoga, Qigong, Tai Chi, and walking in nature. See for more information about healing adrenal fatigue.

MAKE EXERCISE FUN

Don't let exercise become just one more chore to do every day. Make it fun. Change-up your exercise routine regularly to keep it from becoming monotonous. Try something new like joining a class at a local gym. You can also support your favorite charity and enter walking and running events. Better yet, invite a friend to join you. Having an exercise partner will also provide support for the days that you find it challenging to exercise.

Now that you see the benefits that come with regular exercise, it is time to act. Make a decision to exercise regularly. Schedule time to exercise, don't leave it to chance. Exercise is likely the natural stress relief solution you have been looking for. It is now up to you to take action. And remember, make it fun!

CHAPTER 10 – NUTRITION FOR STRESS RELIEF

"We must be willing to let go of the life we planned so as to have the life that is waiting for us."

- Joseph Campbell

Often-times we forget about good health practices and we continue to maintain our busy and hectic lifestyle. Poor food choices rule, as we sacrifice our health by eating fast food. Even worse is the fact that sometimes we just skip eating altogether. This type of lifestyle makes us vulnerable to the effects of stress.

Good nutrition is key for managing and healing stress. Food provides the raw material that the body needs to repair and heal from the effects of stress.

Did you know that 61% of Americans buy food that is highly processed? The standard American diet, also known as SAD, consists of unhealthy fats, refined carbohydrates, and is high in sugars. [16]   How sad is SAD? There is very little nutritional value in a hamburger, French fries, and a soda.

Sometimes, we eat to mask the emotional pain that we feel inside. This is often driven by anxiety and fear. When we eat unconsciously, we make poor, but convenient food choices that ultimately cost us our good health.

If you find yourself stressed out or full of anxiety on a regular basis, then it is time to choose a healthy diet. Now we will go over foods that will make a huge difference in your health.

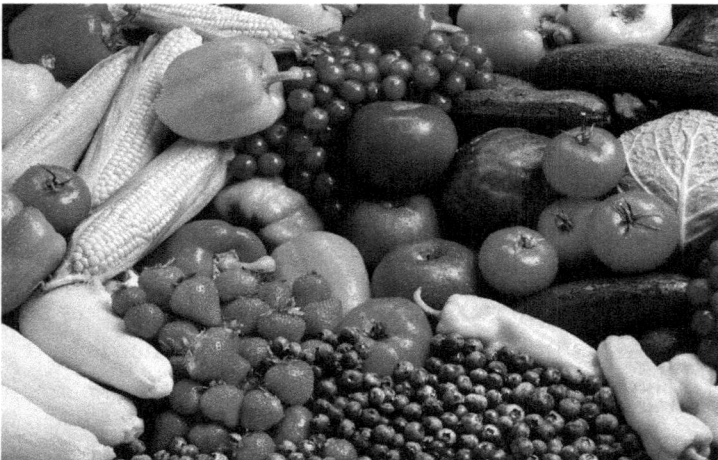

NUTS AND SEEDS

Nuts and seeds are healthy and tasty options that can be taken on the go and eaten as a snack or as a crunchy topping on a salad. Nuts and seeds are full of good fats, protein, vitamins, and minerals. For example, almonds are a good source of Vitamins like B2 and E, both of which are important for the production of serotonin, which is the neurotransmitter that induces a sensation of well-being. They also contain magnesium and zinc. Magnesium is important for proper muscle function and relaxation. Zinc is important for boosting the immune system.

VEGETABLES AND FRUIT

Vegetables in the form of complex carbohydrates are rich in vitamins, minerals, antioxidants, fiber, and water. This means they are a great source of nutrients for supporting and relieving stress. Leafy green vegetables, like kale and spinach, are great sources of vitamins A, C and K, calcium, and fiber. [17] Orange and yellow colored vegetables like carrots, sweet potatoes, peppers, and pumpkin are a great source of vitamins A and C, beta-carotene, flavonoids, lycopene, and potassium. [18]

Fruit are also abundant in vitamins, minerals, antioxidants, fiber, and water. However, since chronic stress can lead to big blood sugar swings, fruit should be limited during stressful events. This is especially true if you have adrenal fatigue.

Eating five servings of fresh vegetables and fruit each day is essential for being healthy and handling stressful situations. It is recommended to eat a mixture of vegetables and fruits of different colors. Fruits and vegetables that are high in fiber help to lower cholesterol levels. [18]

HEALTHY FATS

Healthy fats or essential fatty acids (EFAs) are important for controlling inflammation, which is caused by stress. Healthy fats include both plant-based sources and sea-food based sources. Good sources of healthy fats include coconut oil, flax seeds, hemp seeds, other nuts and seeds, avocado, extra virgin olive oil, and wild salmon (not farm raised). One word of caution is that you should make sure that the oils you are using are not rancid. Monitor the expiration date and store them as described on the labels. Avoid animal based fats (toxins typically collect in the fat of animals) and artificial or processed fats like trans fats (worst type of fat).

WHOLE GRAINS

Whole grains should be included in a healthy diet. They contain lots of vitamins, minerals, fiber, amino acids, and carbohydrates needed for energy production in the body. Healthy whole grains include wheat, brown rice, oats, barley, quinoa, amaranth, and spelt. Avoid gluten-containing grains if you have either a gluten sensitivity or a gluten allergy. Also, avoid processed grains, such as bleached white flour and white rice.

PROTEIN

Protein is essential for muscle and other tissue repair in the body. For those under stress, protein also provides an energy source that does not fluctuate like simple carbohydrates and sugars do, thus avoiding a sugar energy crash. Good food sources of protein are meat, fish, eggs, dairy, nuts and seeds, beans and rice, broccoli, soy, and other plant-based sources.

NUTRITIONAL SUPPLEMENTS

It is important to understand that even if you avoid junk food and eat only organic whole food, that you still may not get enough nutrients from your food. There are many reasons for this. Stress decreases proper digestion, thus while you may be eating adequately, you may not be able to absorb or assimilate the nutrients from the food you eat.

Poor food choices and their acidity may result in an increase in bad bacteria, fungus, and Candida in our gastrointestinal tract, thus leaving us vulnerable to leaky gut syndrome. Therefore, it is important to add supplementation to our daily diet to fill in the gaps caused by eating poor quality food and living with chronic stress.

Better yet, eat higher quality, nutrient-dense food and take a multiple vitamin and mineral supplement. It is important to point out that when you are under stress, your body's nutritional needs increase. Adding proper supplementation will help to reduce the effects of stress. When choosing a supplement, it is important to read the labels. If you find that a supplement has lots of additives, just leave it alone. Whole food based supplements are typically the best ones.

Vitamin A

Vitamin A is crucial for relieving stress. Stress reduces or suppresses healing and repair functions of the body, so it is important to supplement Vitamin A. Natural sources of vitamin A include carrots, sweet potatoes, mangoes, and kale. Since vitamin A is fat soluble, it is best to take vitamin A supplement with fats like olive oil or coconut oil, to name a few. [19]

Vitamin C

Natural and supplemental forms of Vitamin C are crucial for preventing and relieving stress. It is best to get Vitamin C with bioflavonoids, which are plant-based compounds that provide antioxidant effects. [51] The adrenal glands, otherwise known as the stress glands, uses the greatest percentage (approximately 70%) of Vitamin C than any other organ in the body. Vitamin C also prevents the release of stress hormones, like cortisol, thus reducing or preventing a stress response. [20]

Natural sources of vitamin C include papayas, kiwis, goji berries, citrus fruit, camu camu, strawberries, raspberries, cranberries, blueberries, tomatoes, and broccoli, to name a few. [21][52][53] Supplementation is good when food sources are not available. Also, some vitamin C supplements have a time-release form so that vitamin C is released in smaller amounts over time so that it is available to the body. Non-time release forms are also good, but because vitamin C is not stored in the body and is water soluble, excess amounts will be excreted in urine. Therefore, when taking non-time release forms, take smaller amounts more frequently throughout the day for best results.

Vitamin B Complex

Vitamin B complex contains coenzymes necessary for metabolic energy production. It is also important for a healthy nervous system. Since it is water soluble, taking huge amounts at one time will just get you expensive urine, unless the supplement is in a time released formula. Vitamin B complex contains a full spectrum of B vitamins including B1 (thiamine), B2 (riboflavin), B3 (pantothenic acid), niacin (nicotinamide), B6 (pyridoxine), folic acid (folate), B12 (cyanocobalamin), and biotin. Natural sources of B vitamins include meat, eggs, whole grains, leafy green vegetables, legumes, and yeast to name a few. Vitamin B3 is crucial for healing adrenal fatigue caused by stress. Therapeutic doses of vitamin B3 for adrenal fatigue is 500 mg three times a day.

Zinc

Zinc is a trace mineral that is important for cellular metabolism, protein synthesis, and healthy immune function. It is easily depleted when we are under chronic stress. Good food sources of zinc are seafood, meat, legumes, nuts, wheat germ, and yeast. It is important to take zinc with vitamin C, since vitamin C enhances absorption of zinc. [22]

Magnesium

Magnesium contributes to many physiological functions of the body including muscle relaxation. Thus, magnesium is important for relieving stress. Good food sources of magnesium include milk, dairy, whole grains, nuts, legumes, and leafy green vegetables. When taking supplements, it is best to get a magnesium supplement in a glycinate or chelate form with a dose of 200 mg. Take an hour before going to bed. [23] One word of caution is that if you take too much magnesium at one time, it may give you diarrhea or other intestinal issues.

Antioxidants

Normal metabolic processes in the body produce chemicals called free radicals. Free radicals cause cellular oxidation which damages cells and tissues. Some food and supplements that we consume have a protective effect against free radicals and they are called antioxidants. Unfortunately, stress can lead to more free radical production and reduced digestion, which can reduce the amount of antioxidants we assimilate. So, it is crucial to increase our consumption of food and supplements that are high in antioxidants when we are going through a stressful time.

Good food sources of antioxidants include fresh vegetables like leafy greens, tomatoes, and carrots. Fresh fruit is also high in antioxidants, including but not limited to kiwi, goji berries, blueberries, grapes, oranges, cranberries, and raspberries. Other food sources of antioxidants include nuts, herbs and spices, and green tea. Supplement sources of antioxidants include, but are not limited to, vitamin A, vitamin E, vitamin C, selenium, CoQ10, alpha lipoic acid, resveratrol, astaxanthin, and glutathione. [24]

Probiotics

Probiotics are the good bacteria in our intestinal tract. They are responsible for providing balance and when present in adequate numbers they prevent "bad bacteria" and fungi from growing out of control. Thus, probiotics support healthy digestion and elimination in the gastrointestinal tract. Some clinical studies also suggest that taking probiotics can have a positive effect on stress and anxiety. [25] When taking probiotic supplements, it is important to use one that has at least ten bacterial strains (more is better) and fifty billion cultures. [26] Fermented foods are best food sources of probiotics. These include yogurt (unsweetened is best), kimchi, sauerkraut, miso, and kombucha. However, food sources may not provide enough of the good bacteria that is needed if your bad bacteria or fungi are dominant, in which case you will need to supplement.

Digestive Enzymes

Proper digestion is critical for preventing most disease, and it is very critical for preventing and relieving stress. Stress depletes key nutrients for supporting a healthy body, including but not limited to the endocrine system and immune system. That is why supplementing with digestive enzymes are so important.

It starts with supporting the proper amount of acid in the stomach for the digestion where food, especially protein, is broken down. Supplementing with betaine will help provide additional acid if your acid production is low. You can also take some organic apple cider vinegar, which is a natural source of acid. Typically, you can tell if your acid production is low if you get heartburn or indigestion regularly. It is thought that heartburn and indigestion can be caused by too much acid in the stomach. And this can happen if you are drinking a lot of cola and eating food with a lot of tomatoes or with a lot of acid. However, in some cases, it is really an issue with the food not being broken down enough. The next time you get heartburn or indigestion if you take a table spoon of apple cider vinegar and it goes away in a short period of time, then you are not producing enough acid.

Another level of digestion occurs in the small intestine with enzymes produced primarily in the pancreas and small intestines. Supplementing with digestive enzymes for protein (protease), carbohydrates (amylase), and fats (lipase) may be necessary to support proper assimilation of nutrients in the small intestine for those that may not be producing enough on your own. One sign that you may need to supplement with digestive enzymes is if you produce a lot of gas following a meal. [27]

L-Glutamine

L-Glutamine is an amino acid present in the body. It can help to increase your energy, support the intestines, boost immune function, stabilize blood sugar, and increase the production of growth hormones. It also helps to reduce stomach ulcers. It is recommended to take between 1 to 5 grams per day. [28] You can find L-Glutamine at any health food or nutrition store.

PROPER HYDRATION

Getting adequate amounts of pure water is important for proper hydration. If stress is chronic for too long, the adrenal glands may become fatigued to the point that they can no longer produce sufficient amounts of hormones. While these hormones are typically referred to as stress hormones, small amounts are necessary for normal body functions and to adapt to physical and mental exertions.

One of the hormones produced by the adrenal glands, aldosterone, is responsible for water and sodium re-absorption and retention in the kidneys. Thus if aldosterone is low due to adrenal fatigue, then we can become dehydrated. It is important to balance water and electrolytes for proper hydration. It is recommended to drink half your weight in ounces of water. Therefore, if you weighed 100 lbs., then you would drink 50 ounces of water daily for proper hydration. If your aldosterone production is low, you may find it beneficial to mix your water with a pinch of pink or Celtic sea salt.

FOODS TO AVOID

It is best to eliminate all heavily processed food, including white flour and sugar. It is also best to avoid food that has additives, preservatives, and artificial food coloring. It is important to read the food labels to understand what is included in food products. If you don't recognize the ingredients, then it is best not to eat the food. Ingredients that should be avoided include monosodium glutamate (MSG), nitrites, nitrates, high fructose corn syrup, trans fats, food coloring, and artificial sweeteners.

And it is important to avoid caffeine since it adds more stress to your body due to its stimulating effect (hard on the adrenals) and it can dehydrate you since it is a diuretic (enhances water elimination through urination), especially if you don't drink enough water.

CHAPTER 11 – HOLISTIC REMEDIES FOR STRESS RELIEF

"If opportunity doesn't knock, build a door."

- Milton Berle

Medications are often prescribed for relieving stress and anxiety. However, most of these medications come with a long list of side effects. It is important to note that there are natural, effective, and holistic remedies for managing and relieving the effects of stress, without side effects. Each remedy has their own unique characteristics for relieving stress.

BACH FLOWER ESSENCES

Bach Flower Essence are natural herbal remedies made of flower essences that have unique subtle energies for bringing balance to specific negative emotional states and moods. There are 38 different flower essences. Each one corresponds to a specific emotional state, like anxiety, stress, and depression. There is also one popular remedy, "Rescue Remedy", that has a combination of flower essences that provides relief for acute emotions and moods. Here's a small sampling of some popular essences. [29]

Cherry Plum can be used when you have a fear of losing control, going mad, or acting irrationally.

Aspen is used when you have a fear that can't be identified, like a general feeling of anxiety or a feeling that something bad is going to happen.

Elm is useful when you feel overwhelmed with too many responsibilities.

Impatiens helps you when you feel frustrated, irritable, and impatient.

Larch is useful when you lack the confidence to do something.

ADAPTOGENS FOR STRESS RELIEF

Adaptogens are plants or herbs that have compounds that help the body cope with stress whether physical, psychological, or even environmental. They act to bring balance to the mechanisms that they affect.

Ashwagandha

Ashwagandha (also known as Withania Somnifera, winter cherry, or poison gooseberry) is one of the most important plant medicines in Ayurvedic therapy. Recent studies have proved Ashwagandha's restorative role in stress reduction, mood elevation, and improving brain function. One study showed that Ashwagandha also helps by boosting up the levels of a key compound within brain cells responsible for the protection of these cells against aging and damage by stress. [30] Also, Ashwagandha acts like a potent antioxidant that may protect brains cells against the damaging effects of our modern lifestyle, including the effects of stress. [31]

In a clinical trial of humans, researchers observed the effects of ashwagandha extract in a condition of elevated cortisol (stress hormone) level. Higher levels of cortisol are thought to be responsible for many of the adverse effects of stress. The results of this study were very positive as the participants reported reduced fatigue, better sleep, increased energy, and sense of well-being. Improvements in other measurable parameters including a reduction of cortisol levels (up to 26%), improved lipid profiles, and a decline in fasting blood sugar level (in diabetic subjects) was also observed in these patients. This study also proposed the use of this remedy in addressing many of the psychological and health issues that are common today. [32]

Astragalus

Astragalus is a herb that is indigenous in China, where it is known as *"huang qi"*. Astragalus root is an adaptogenic herb that is effective at relieving the effects of stress. Astragalus is also known for activating the immune system. [33] This explains why this herb is used to supplement some cancer remedies such as chemotherapy.

This herb has also been shown to improve the cardiovascular system thus reducing the chances of congestive heart failure and myocardial infarction (heart attack). [34] Finally, the herb functions by enhancing the activity of the vital organs such as the liver and the kidneys by increasing the blood flow. [35] Astragalus root is often taken as a decoction after boiling it in water. Also, the root can be dried and ground into a powder that is placed into capsules.

Lemon Balm

Lemon Balm, also known as Melissa Officinalis, is an herb belonging to the mint family that relieves anxiety, muscle tension, stress, and insomnia. [36][37] Lemon balm has been shown to be effective for controlling stress in as little as 15 days. [38] It is also used for other problems such as Alzheimer's disease, high blood pressure, insomnia, lack of appetite, skin problems, insect bites, pain relief, and tumors.

It is commonly used for relief of menstrual symptoms, infant colic issues, and irritable bowel syndrome. [39]

Lemon balm also contains flavonoids that enhance antioxidant activity, which promotes the repair of damaged cells. Lemon balm is available in different forms including dried leaves, capsules, tinctures, tea, extracts, and oils.

Licorice Root

Licorice root is an herb that has many benefits including stress relief. Licorice root is known for its effects on the body including boosting the immune system, healing ulcers, relieving pain, relieving stress, acting as an expectorant, and relaxing bronchial spasms. [40]

It has also been used for its anti-inflammatory properties in Traditional Chinese medicine for centuries. [41] Research has also shown that licorice root is beneficial for managing adrenal fatigue. Check out for more information about how licorice root can help with adrenal fatigue. Licorice root is also beneficial for reducing the symptoms of chronic fatigue and fibromyalgia. [40]

Rhodiola Rosea

Rhodiola has long been used in Europe and Asia for boosting energy and reducing mental fatigue. [42] Rhodiola Rosea has been studied for its effects of preventing fatigue and stress, and its antioxidant effects. It is also known for boosting immune function and improving sexual energy. It is best to take Rhodiola early in the day since it can interfere with sleep. [43]

Rhodiola's ability to relieve stress is attributed to its ability to bring balance to the body through enhancing serotonin, norepinephrine, and endorphins in the brain. This results in a calming effect and improved cognitive function. More recent research has shown that Rhodiola acts as a strong antioxidant that protects the nervous system from oxidative stress. [42]

Panax Ginseng

Panax Ginseng, also known as Asian or Korean Ginseng, is known in Asia for its adaptogenic effects on the body. Studies have shown Panax Ginseng to improve mood and calmness. It has been found to reduce adrenal fatigue and boost the immune system. Other studies show that it has anti-inflammatory properties. It is recommended to take 500 mg twice daily for stress, tension, or fatigue. [44]

Panax Ginseng is known in Traditional Chinese Medicine (TCM) to have a yang energy quality, making it a good tonic for colder climates. It is best prepared in tea form by cooking the ginseng root in a slow cooker for about eight hours or over night. This was prescribed to me by a doctor of TCM and it was quite effective at boosting my energy level.

AROMATHERAPY

Aromatherapy is the use of aromatic plant-based oils, referred to as essential oils, for improving one's health and well-being. When the oils are inhaled, they immediately interact with the brain to elicit a desired response. These essential oils can be used in massage oil, in a diffuser, they can be applied topically, and they can be inhaled. For stress relief, it is important to use essential oils that are calming, relaxing, and soothing. Essential oils that are typically used for stress relief include peppermint, lavender, jasmine, chamomile, and lemongrass. [45]

CHAPTER 12 – STEPS TO REDUCE STRESS IN YOUR RELATIONSHIPS

"No matter how hard the past, you can always begin again."

- Buddha

Life can be very difficult when there is stress in a relationship. There are many reasons for feeling stress in a relationship including, financial issues, disagreements over how to discipline the kids, working too much, health problems, miscommunication, and many more. You may be wondering what you should do when there is stress in your relationship. Here's a few things you can do to find stress relief in your relationship.

IDENTIFY YOUR DISAGREEMENTS

The first step to handling a disagreement is to be explicit about what the disagreement is. Write down a list of ideas about that which you both disagree and is the source of your stress. Make sure you capture both sides of the disagreement. Whatever seems to feel most threatening, put it on the list.

WRITE DOWN THE REASONS FOR THE DISAGREEMENTS

Write down the reasons you disagree with each individual challenge on the list. Clearly understand what the conflict is for each of you. The clearer you understand the conflict details, the more effectively you can resolve the conflict and reduce stress.

REMEMBER LOVE

Before you get into another argument, commit to remembering that you love each other. Remember how special your relationship is. Your relationship is worth the effort to find a solution. Therefore, you must have compassion and see the other's point of view. Forgiveness and compromise are key to finding a solution to your disagreement and your stress. It is important to reflect on the positive moments in your life. Express gratitude for the fact that the person is a part of your life.

ACKNOWLEDGE YOUR EFFORT

Acknowledge the amount of effort that the both of you are putting into resolving the differences, even if you haven't found a solution. Disclaiming either of your efforts to resolve the situation may result in another disagreement. Families that made it through *"The Great Depression"* did so by remembering to love one another and finding ways to just deal with the challenges.

BE POSITIVE

It is important to be positive while working towards a solution to your relationship problems. Focus on the good in your relationship. Oftentimes we get stuck on some negative aspect which is only a very small part of the relationship. That means that most of the relationship is positive. Focus on the positive. Express your gratitude for the positive aspects of your relationship. Be kind and generous in your relationships. This is the key to reduce tension and stress in your relationships.

CHAPTER 13 – PREVENTING STRESS

"Do not anticipate trouble or worry about what may never happen. Keep in the sunlight."

- Benjamin Franklin

Ultimately, we should live life without being consumed and overwhelmed by stress. We should be able to adapt to changes and challenges in life without becoming stressed out. The ideas in this chapter will help you to prevent stress from happening in the first place. Now with that said, will you be able to completely eliminate stress from your life, probably not. That is because we are humans and we aren't perfect. We have feelings and emotions and we have been programmed with struggles since our birth. And there are things that happen that we can't control, like natural disasters. However, we can still strive to prevent stress as much as possible.

HAVE AN OPEN MIND

One way to prevent stress is to have an open mind. This means to be more open to new ideas and new situations. When we become resistant to new things because we fear that we may get hurt in some way, we become stuck in our past experiences. This perception will cause all new situations to become stressful before they even happen. Again, this is wasting our present moments worrying about some future event that will likely not happen the way we are negatively imagining it. This negativity is triggered by our fears. Instead, have an open mind and look at new experience as an adventure. When presented with a new situation, ask yourself, "What exciting thing will I learn this time?" When you have an open mind and you change your perspective to a positive one, you will find that life will become a whole lot less stressful.

TAKE A MENTAL TIMEOUT

When things in life start to move too fast and you start to feel overwhelmed, take a mental timeout. What I mean is to simply take a break. Find a place where you can get away for a short time to let your mind rest. Life can become overwhelming when we try to juggle too many tasks at once, whether it is voluntary or out of obligation. Take a mental timeout from the chaos. There are many things you can do for the timeout. You could take a walk in nature, exercise, meditate, or talk to a friend. Don't wait for a full blown stress crisis to move you to action. If you take the timeout in the beginning, it will calm your mind so that you can get a better perspective on things.

SET BOUNDARIES

It is important to know your limitations and set boundaries so that you don't over-extend yourself. Be realistic and set the boundaries ahead of time, so you know when you've reached your limit. For instance, if you already have two projects that you are working on at the same time and you know that you don't have time for anything else, then set boundaries so that you won't take on any new projects until you complete the ones you are working on. Don't be afraid to speak up and say NO if someone asks you to work on something else. Another type of boundary is that you know you must eat at a certain time or you will get weak. So, don't let anyone at work talk you into working over when you know you need to eat to prevent yourself from getting weak or sick. I recommend creating a boundaries card and write down boundaries that are important for you to keep. Write down your response to someone if they ask you to do something beyond your boundary. This way there will be less chance of someone talking you into doing something you really don't want to do. Stick to your boundaries and let people know that they aren't flexible.

PLAN FOR STRESSFUL EVENTS

We don't always know in advance when stressful events will show up in our lives, but sometimes we do. In these cases, we can plan ahead so that we know how to handle the situation. This will help to reduce our stress over the event. For example, if you know that in a week you need to give a presentation at work, then you start working on it right away to make it the best presentation ever. You can start by creating an outline of the topic you will be presenting. Next, you can create a slide presentation based on the outline. Then, you can practice the presentation at home or with another colleague to fine tune it. Planning and being prepared for events that we know are coming will reduce the pressure when the big day arrives.

DEVELOP YOUR INTUITION

Your intuition is that gut feeling that tells you when something is right or wrong. It's your intuition that tells you to go a different direction and you avoid an accident, for example. When you are just starting to develop your intuition, you may wonder how to tell the difference from your intuition and your overactive imagination. It takes practice. Over time you will learn the subtle signs that indicate if it is from your intuition. One way to tell is that some information comes to you out of the blue, not from some logical and rational thought process. Trusting in your intuition will help you to avoid some stressful situations.

TALK IT OUT

Sometimes, it helps to talk to someone about what you are feeling before it becomes too stressful. Getting another person's perspective on your situation can help to prevent you from misinterpreting or exaggerating a situation. Another person's perspective is especially important if they have experience dealing with the situation that you are facing. Sometimes we just need to blow off a little steam. In this case, find someone that you know is a good listener.

FIND YOUR PASSION

Find something to do that you are passionate about. Maybe there is a hobby that you've always wanted to try. Maybe you've always wanted to learn ballroom dancing. How about taking an art class? Sometimes when we go through the motions of life, we forget about what we are truly passionate about because we need to work to pay the bills. If you are stressed, it is a good sign that you have lost your passion for life. If you don't exactly know what you are passionate about, take a risk, be courageous, and try something new. Trying new things will help you to bring passion back into your life.

GET A HEALTH AND WELLNESS COACH

If you find yourself with a health issue, like needing to lose weight, wanting to improve your eating habits, or wanting to reduce stress, and you don't know the best way to handle it, you could turn to a health and wellness coach. A health and wellness coach looks at health from a holistic perspective, which includes mind, body, spirit, environment, relationships, and passion to name a few. They will help to guide you towards your desired goal, but you must put in the time and do the work.

Let's say you want to learn how to relax more. A coach would help you find options to bring peace and relaxation into your life. A good coach will help you to see the best way to integrate the solution into your life so it becomes part of your routine, like brushing your teeth. Seek out a health and wellness coach before your health issue becomes a source of stress for you. They will help you along your journey to your desired outcome.

SPEND QUALITY TIME WITH FAMILY AND FRIENDS

The key to a long and healthy life is to surround yourself with loving family and friends regularly. Spending quality time with them is important to you and them. You are there for each other, to support each other, to have fun together, and to help each other through tough times. I recommend that you invite them to join you in some of the stress relief and prevention techniques discussed in this book. Life is more enjoyable when you can share it with the ones you love.

CHAPTER 14 – HEALING ADRENAL FATIGUE

"Don't let your mind bully your body into believing it must carry the burden of its worries."

\- Astrid Alauda

The adrenal glands are two very small glands that sit on top of the kidneys. They are responsible for managing normal wake cycle, managing blood sugar levels, sodium and water balance, sexual function, and stress adaptation. [46]

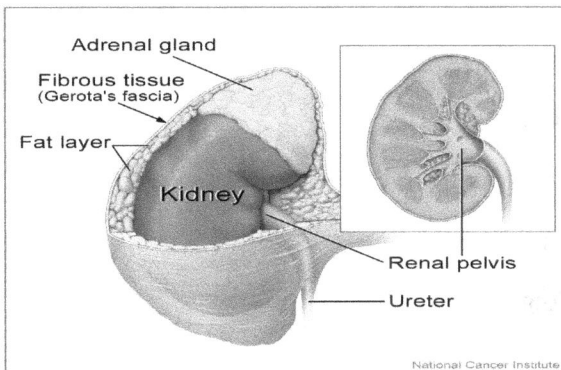

Public Domain Image, Courtesy of National Cancer Institute

77

ADRENAL FATIGUE

While stress is typically accompanied by high levels of hormones produced by the adrenal gland, in extreme cases the adrenals can become fatigued, in which case, they don't produce enough hormones. It is important to point out that cortisol, one of the hormones produced by the adrenal glands, is needed in normal amounts for basic cellular function and to manage normal levels of inflammation in the body due to normal metabolic activities.

When the adrenal glands are fatigued, due to long-term chronic stress, they are depleted and produce lower amounts of the hormones, which can cause serious health issues if left unmanaged.

Symptoms of Adrenal Fatigue

◆ Mental and physical fatigue

◆ Mental fog

◆ Poor memory

◆ Inflammation

◆ Muscular weakness

◆ Weight loss

◆ Low blood pressure

◆ Inability to adapt and deal with normal stresses and major stress events

◆ Electrolyte imbalances

I know from personal experience the debilitating effects of adrenal fatigue and that's why it is so important to seek out proper treatment from a qualified holistic health doctor. With that said, I will present some information here for educational purposes that you can discuss with your doctor to see if they are right for your situation. Remember, everyone is different and the causes of illness and the treatments of illness are individual as well.

It is important to also understand that body fatigue can be caused by health issues other than adrenal fatigue. For instance, if your thyroid is under functioning, it will cause your metabolism to slow down and you may become sluggish or fatigued. So, it is important to have both thyroid and adrenal gland hormone levels tested.

One word of caution is that most traditional Western medical doctors do not accept that the adrenals can be fatigued. They feel that the only disease states of the adrenals are that they produce too much hormones, which is the case with Cushing's syndrome, or they produce too little hormones, which is the case with Addison's disease. However, doctors and practitioners of natural and integrative medicine are finding that this is not the case.

There are saliva tests that can be taken that can show the level of cortisol over time, which may be between the two extremes. The test results along with the patient's history can establish enough information to diagnose adrenal fatigue.

REVERSING ADRENAL FATIGUE

Adrenal fatigue can be managed, and even be "cured" or reversed through eating a proper diet, taking necessary supplements, getting adequate amounts of rest and sleep, and by changing your lifestyle. Let's go through each of these to understand what can be done.

Eating a "proper" diet is critical for healing adrenal fatigue. The information presented in is a great place to start for understanding the components of the proper diet for healing adrenal fatigue. I will go over some things that are really important under the context of dealing with adrenal fatigue. First, it can't be stated enough that you should eliminate all processed and refined food. You can't heal adrenal fatigue on a Standard American Diet (SAD).

Eating fresh vegetables, fruit, and whole grains are important. If you have lots of blood sugar swings (typical with adrenal fatigue), it is advisable to limit the amount of fruit and other very sweet carbohydrates, which could make the swings worse. Also, getting adequate amounts of protein are critical to stabilizing the blood sugar and preventing muscle weakness. This is especially important if you are vegan and are not eating animal based food. Foods and supplements that are high in vitamin C are necessary to support the revitalization of the adrenal glands, since they are the largest consumer of vitamin C in the body.

Supplementation is important to provide raw nutrients for the healing of the adrenal glands and to manage the symptoms associated with the weakness until the adrenals are rejuvenated. B vitamins and in particular Pantothenic Acid (vitamin B5) is very important for reducing fatigue. You can start with 1000 mcg of B5 and gradually increase to 1000 mcg of B5 three times a day.

Supplementation with vitamin C, as we have mentioned, is very important for rebuilding the adrenal glands. Vitamin C is best taken with bioflavonoids, in amounts of 1000 mg, which can be gradually increased over time. Therapeutic doses of vitamin C range from 2,000 mg to 5,000 mg for managing adrenal fatigue. Stop increasing the dose of vitamin C when your stool is like diarrhea. Then, you can back off by 1000 mg. [47] Magnesium will help for muscle fatigue, muscle cramps and stiffness, depression, and insomnia. Taking 400 mg per day is recommended. Probiotics are important to assist in digestion, which is often poor in those with stress related illnesses. [48]

One herbal remedy that I have found particularly beneficial is licorice root extract. Licorice root is crucial for people with low cortisol production. At a given time, whatever cortisol is not immediately used, it is broken down and eliminated. For someone that has adrenal fatigue, it is important to keep as much cortisol as possible. Licorice root blocks the breakdown of cortisol. [49]

I have personally found that liquid licorice root extract is best because it is easy to take and easy to digest. However, for those people that have high blood pressure, you should consult your doctor before taking licorice root, since it may cause an increase in blood pressure and should be monitored. Licorice root also has an anti-inflammatory effect.

Another supplement that I have found helpful is L-Tyrosine. L-Tyrosine is an amino acid that is more known for its utilization by the thyroid and thyroid hormone production. However, L-Tyrosine is also a building block of the adrenal glands. It is recommended to take L-Tyrosine on an empty stomach before breakfast in the morning.

If your aldosterone levels are low (get tested to find out), you may find it helpful to take a teaspoon of sea salt in warm water first thing in the morning. It will help to replenish your depleted sodium levels.

Proper rest and sleep are also critical for healing adrenal fatigue. Physical exertion also causes the adrenal glands to produce cortisol. So, it is important not to over work yourself and not to over exercise. Less is better when adrenal fatigue is concerned. Take things slow and get proper rest after exercising or doing physical labor.

Getting the proper amount of sleep is also important. First, going to bed early and consistently is important. Staying up late with a "second wind" will only utilize more cortisol than necessary, thus taking a toll on already fatigued adrenal glands. When you do this, you may find that it is more difficult to get up the next morning and you may feel very tired or fatigued than if you hadn't stayed up too late. Make sure you get at least eight hours of sleep. Also, sleeping in occasionally will help to recharge your adrenals.

Lifestyle modification is important when dealing with adrenal fatigue. You must recognize that the reason your adrenals are fatigued is due to living with chronic stress over a long period of time. So, if you want to heal your adrenal glands you must get a handle of your stress. Lucky for you, that is the topic of this book and you will benefit from the information in this book for dealing with stress. I suggest starting with understanding the sources of your stress.

FOOD AND ENVIRONMENTAL ALLERGIES

Allergies can also place a heavy burden on the adrenal glands. If you have food and/or environmental allergies, then you need to take extra precautions to alleviate or prevent additional complications of adrenal fatigue. Food allergies mean that you need to pay close attention to the food ingredients and pesticides. Avoid any food allergens at all costs. If you suspect an allergen but you are not sure which food that is causing your symptoms, then you can try to eliminate a food type for a couple of weeks and then reintroduce it slowly. If your symptoms improve after elimination and then get worse after reintroducing the food, then it may be best to avoid this food. You can eliminate other foods one-by-one to see if there are allergenic foods in your diet.

One thing to consider is that depending on the manufacturing practices, some food may be cross-contaminated during the manufacturing processing of food. I have a gluten allergy and found this out the hard way. Some manufacturing equipment that processes wheat, for example, may also process other grains, like oats. Oats don't have gluten, naturally, however, they can be cross-contaminated during the manufacturing process. Typically, the food packaging will mention if the food was processed in a facility that also processes known allergens like wheat or gluten. For oatmeal, you can look for certified gluten-free oats. This is one of many types of allergens. Seek out professional medical consultation if you have questions.

Environmental allergies are caused by allergens in our environment like tree pollen, pollution, toxic cleaning supplies, new product and carpet out-gassing, perfumes and colognes, second-hand smoke, and many other chemicals that are either natural or manufactured. It is important to avoid environmental allergies as much as possible. For products that you use regularly, look for non-toxic versions, like natural plant-based cleaning supplies. Dust is also a source of allergies. So, it is important to vacuum and dust regularly. Get a good air purifier, preferably one that has a high-efficiency particulate arrestance (HEPA) filter, which eliminates 99.97% of air particles that have a size of 0.3 micrometers in size. [54]

Keep in mind that allergies, whether food or environmental in nature, are individual in nature. It is important to do all you can to strengthen your immune system through proper diet, exercise, and eliminating allergens. Everyone is different. If you find it difficult to identify the source of your allergies, you can seek out a qualified health care practitioner for allergy testing.

GET TESTED

The best way to know whether your adrenal glands are weak or fatigued is by thoroughly examining your symptoms, your history, and your test results. First, your doctor should ask you about your current symptoms, your past behaviors, including stress, diet, and sleep habits, to name a few. Then, they will recommend a test to measure your adrenal hormone levels.

As I have stated previously, standard medical blood tests don't often identify adrenal fatigue because of the traditional medical biases against the existence of the condition. I have found that an adrenal stress test involving the collection of saliva four times in a day to be quite effective at identifying the condition and at identifying when I have recovered.

Seek out a qualified holistic health practitioner for providing the test kit and interpreting the results. I have used the *"Adrenal Stress Index Panel"* by DiagnosTechs, as recommended by my holistic health doctor, and have found it very beneficial for identifying my adrenal weakness and for monitoring my progress throughout my treatment. [50]

CHAPTER 15 – CONCLUSION

"If the problem can be solved why worry? If the problem cannot be solved worrying will do you no good."

- Santideva

I hope that you have benefited from the information presented in this book. In the previous chapters, we covered how stress affects the body and the mind. You saw that the brain and the adrenal glands play an important role for adapting to stress through the production of neurotransmitters and hormones. And you also saw how chronic stress causes health issues when they are not properly dealt with.

Effective strategies for managing and preventing stress were also presented. It is about making informed choices and modifying your lifestyle to better handle stress.

You learned about nutrition and holistic remedies for stress relief. You also learned about handling stress in your relationships. And you learned how to recognize and manage adrenal fatigue.

There are so many options when it comes to managing and relieving stress. So now, it is up to you to make a choice to live as stress-free a life as you can. I recommend that you start out by choosing one or two options presented in the previous chapters and find the best ways to integrate them into your life.

It only takes small steps to begin to experience the benefits. Then later you can gradually add other techniques and options that will further improve your chances for living a stress-free life. Be patient and creative. But most importantly, take action to reduce and eliminate the stress in your life. You can make a difference. You can heal stress.

If you would like help to relieve or prevent stress, check out http://www.EliminateStressNow.com.

FROM THE AUTHOR

First of all, thank you for purchasing this book *"Healing Stress."* While you could have picked any number of books to read, you picked this one, and for that, I am very grateful.

I hope that it added value to your everyday life. If so, it would be nice if you would share this book with your family and friends by posting to Twitter, Facebook, and other social media.

Also, if you enjoyed this book and found it beneficial, I'd like to hear from you. I hope that you could take some time to post a review. Your feedback and support will greatly help me improve my writing for future projects and make this book even better.

If you would like to leave a review, all you have to do is to click on the following link for the *"Healing Stress"* book page and select the store of your choice; https://books2read.com/HealingStress.

Finally, if you'd like to get notifications of new book releases, special offers, and other related content, please join my email list at https://ivs-publishing.gr8.com/.

REFERENCES

1. *"Cortisol"*, Wikipedia.org. Web Retrieved May 8, 2016 from https://en.wikipedia.org/wiki/Cortisol.

2. Susser MD, Murray. *"Thymus, Stress and Just Being Sick"*. Web Retrieved May 8, 2016 from http://www.murraysussermd.com/thymus-stress-and-just-being-sick/

3. Jenner, Dr. Nicholas. (2014, August 14). *"Stress: where it all starts"*. Web Retrieved May 8, 2016 from https://boundariesofthesoul.com/2012/08/14/stress-where-it-all-starts/

4. *"Stress"*, Research & Clinical Trials for Health Professionals. Web Retrieved May 8, 2016 from http://umm.edu/health/medical/reports/articles/stress.

5. Aldwin, Carolyn M., et. al. (2011). *"Do Stress Trajectories Predict Mortality in Older Men? Longitudinal Findings from the VA Normative Aging Study"* Journal of Aging Research. Web Retrieved May 1, 2016 from http://www.hindawi.com/journals/jar/2011/896109/.

6. *"Women with impaired stress hormone before pregnancy have lower-birthweight babies"*, Science News. Web Retrieved May 01, 2016 from https://www.sciencedaily.com/releases/2016/03/16031810 2118.htm.

7. *"Stress and Sleep"*, American Psychological Association. Web Retrieved May 2, 2016 from http://www.apa.org/news/press/releases/stress/2013/sleep .aspx.

8. *"Social Media and the Cost of Caring"*, Pew Research Center. Web Retrieved May 8, 2016 from http://www.pewinternet.org/2015/01/15/social-media-and-stress/.

9. Gendry, Sebastien. *"Why More Laughter = Less Stress = Better Health And More Energy"*, Laughter Online University. Web Retrieved April 9, 2016 from http://www.laughteronlineuniversity.com/laughter-less-stress-better-health-energy/.

10. *"National Sleep Foundation's sleep time duration recommendations: methodology and results summary"*. Sleep Health Journal, March 2015 Volume 1, Issue 1. Web Retrieved May 5, 2016 from http://www.sleephealthjournal.org/article/S2352-7218%2815%2900015-7/fulltext.

11. *"Insufficient Sleep Is a Public Health Problem"*, CDC. Web Retrieved May 5, 2016 from http://www.cdc.gov/features/dssleep/index.html#References.

12. *"Prescription Sleep Aid Use Among Adults: United States, 2005-2010"*, CDC. Web Retrieved May 5, 2016 from http://www.cdc.gov/nchs/products/databriefs/db127.htm.

13. Thompson, Judy. *"Sleep Your Way to Better Health"*, Laughter Online University. Web Retrieved May 5, 2016 from http://www.arcamax.com/healthandspirit/health/healthtips/s-95808-207008.

14. Carter Psy.D., Sherrie Bourg. (2011, May 27). *"Has Sleep and Stress Become a Vicious Cycle in Your Life?"*, Psychology Today. Web Retrieved May 10, 2016 from https://www.psychologytoday.com/blog/high-octane-women/201105/has-sleep-and-stress-become-vicious-cycle-in-your-life.

15. *"Exercise and stress: Get moving to manage stress"*, Mayo Clinic. Web Retrieved May 6, 2016 from http://www.mayoclinic.org/healthy-lifestyle/stress-management/in-depth/exercise-and-stress/art-20044469.

16. Oaklander, Mandy. (2015, May 21). *"61% of Your Calories Are From Highly Processed Food: Study"*, Time. Web Retrieved April 30, 2016 from http://time.com/3888102/processed-food-sugar-fat/.

17. Nierenberg, Cari. *"Leafy Greens – Ranked and Rated"*, WebMD. Web Retrieved May 7, 2016 from http://www.webmd.com/diet/healthy-kitchen-11/leafy-greens-rated.

18. Stein, Natalie. *"Nutrients in Red and Orange Vegetables"*, LiveStrong.com. Web Retrieved May 7, 2016 from http://www.livestrong.com/article/540938-nutrients-in-red-and-orange-vegetables/.

19. Weil M.D., Andrew, et al. *"Facts About Vitamin A"*, DrWeil.com. Web Retrieved May 7, 2016 from http://www.drweil.com/drw/u/ART02759/facts-about-vitamin-a.

20. *"Vitamin C Reduces Effects Of Chronic Stress"*, Mercola.com. Web Retrieved May 7, 2016 from http://articles.mercola.com/sites/articles/archive/2008/01/02/vitamin-c-reduces-effects-of-chronic-stress.aspx.

21. *"Vitamin C"*. whfoods.org. Web Retrieved May 7, 2016 from http://www.whfoods.com/genpage.php?tname=nutrient&dbid=109.

22. *"How does Stress affect health?"*, Holistic-Back-Relief.com. Web Retrieved May 7, 2016 from http://www.holistic-back-relief.com/how-does-stress-affect-health.html.

23. Bhatia, Dr. Tasneem. *"Supplements That Fight Stress"*, DoctorOz.com. Web Retrieved April 29, 2016 from http://www.doctoroz.com/article/supplements-fight-stress/.

24. *"The Ultimate Guide to Antioxidants"*, Mercola.com. Web Retrieved April 30, 2016 from http://articles.mercola.com/antioxidants.aspx.

25. *"Addressing stress and anxiety with probiotics"*, Nutraceutical Business Review. Web Retrieved May 7, 2016 from http://www.nutraceuticalbusinessreview.com/technical/arti cle_page/Addressing_stress_and_anxiety_with_probiotics/ 103853.

26. *"What Should You Look For In A Probiotic?"*, blog.brendwatson.com. Web Retrieved May 7, 2016 from http://blog.brendawatson.com/forum/frequently-asked-questions/what-should-you-look-for-in-a-probiotic/.

27. Gerstmar, Dr. Tim. *"Everything You Ever Wanted to Know about Digestive Enzymes"*, Whole 9. Web Retrieved April 30, 2016 from http://whole9life.com/2012/09/digestive-enzymes-101/.

28. *"What is L-Glutamine: Uses, Effects, Benefits and Dosages"*, Nootriment. Web Retrieved April 30, 2016 from http://nootriment.com/l-glutamine/.

29. *"Guide to the remedies"*, The Back Centre. Web Retrieved May 8, 2016 from http://www.bachcentre.com/centre/remedies.htm.

30. Baitharu I, Jain V, Deep SN, Shroff S, Sahu JK, Naik PK, et al. *"Withanolide A Prevents Neurodegeneration by Modulating Hippocampal Glutathione Biosynthesis during Hypoxia"*. PLoS ONE. 2014;9(10):e105311.

31. Bhattacharya A, Ghosal S, Bhattacharya SK. *"Antioxidant effect of Withania somnifera glycowithanolides in chronic footshock stress-induced perturbations of oxidative free radical scavenging enzymes and lipid peroxidation in rat frontal cortex and striatum."* Journal of ethnopharmacology. 2001;74(1):1-6.

32. Kiefer, Dale. *"Ashwagandha Stress Reduction, Neural Protection, and a Lot More from an Ancient Herb"*, Life Extension Magazine. Web Retrieved May 1, 2016 from http://www.lifeextension.com/magazine/2006/6/report_as hwa/page-01.

33. *"Astragalus"*, Weil Herbs. Web Retrieved, February 20, 2016 from http://www.drweil.com/drw/u/REM00002/Astragalus-Dr-Weils-Herbal-Remedies.html.

34. Wellness Mama. *"Benefits of Astragalus Root. Retrieved"*. Web Retrieved from 2/10/2016 http://wellnessmama.com/15726/astragalus-root-benefits/.

35. *"10 Proven Benefits of Astragalus Root (#4 Is Vital)"*, Dr. Axe. Web Retrieved, May 8, 2016 from http://draxe.com/astragalus/.

36. Johnson, RN, BSN, Tiesha D. *"Quick Relief from Anxiety and Stress Without Tranquilizer Drugs."* (August 2007). Life Extension Magazine. Web Retrieved, May 8, 2016 from http://www.lifeextension.com/magazine/2007/8/report_str ess_anxiety/page-01.

37. *"How to use Lemon Balm for Anxiety Relief & Memory Improvement"*, Nootriment. Web Retrieved, May 8, 2016 from http://nootriment.com/lemon-balm/.

38. Johnson, RN, BSN, Tiesha D. *"Lemon Balm In Natural Stress Relief"*. TIKVA. Web Retrieved, May 8, 2016 from http://medicalpublications.org/natural-stress-relief/.

39. *"Find a Vitamin or Supplement. Lemon Balm"*, WebMD. Web Retrieved May 8, 2016 from http://www.webmd.com/vitamins-supplements/ingredientmono-437-lemon%20balm.aspx? activeingredientid=437&.

40. *"Licorice Root (Glycyrrhiza Glabra)"*, Herbwisdom.com. Web Retrieved May 14, 2016 from http://www.herbwisdom.com/herb-licorice-root.html.

41. *"Licorice Root Benefits Adrenal Fatigue & Leaky Gut"*, draxe.com. Web Retrieved May 14, 2016 from http://draxe.com/licorice-root/.

42. *"Rhodiola"* (December 2007). Life Extension Magazine. Web Retrieved May 1, 2016 from http://www.lifeextension.com/magazine/2007/12/report_n utraceutical/page-01.

43. *"Rhodiola for What Ails You?"*, drweil.com, Q & A Library. Web Retrieved May 1, 2016 from http://www.drweil.com/drw/u/QAA400399/Rhodiola-for-What-Ails-You.html.

44. *"Ginseng Benefits: Less Stress & Better Brain Function"*, draxe.com. Web Retrieved May 1, 2016 from http://draxe.com/ginseng-benefits/.

45. Group DC NP, Dr Edward, *"Can You Eliminate Stress with Aromatherapy?"*, Global Healing Center. Web Retrieved May 1, 2016 from http://www.globalhealingcenter.com/natural-health/can-you-eliminate-stress-with-aromatherapy/.

46. Craze, Lori Anderson. *"Foods That Heal Adrenal Glands"*, Livestrong.com. Web Retrieved May 1, 2016 from http://www.livestrong.com/article/340770-foods-that-heal-adrenal-glands/.

47. *"Facts about Vitamin C and Adrenal Fatigue"*, AdrenalFatigueRecovery.com. Web Retrieved May 7, 2016 from http://www.adrenalfatiguerecovery.com/vitamin-c.html.

48. Hansen, Fawne, *"Supplements For Adrenal Fatigue"*, The Adrenal Fatigue Solution. Web Retrieved May 1, 2016 from http://adrenalfatiguesolution.com/adrenal-fatigue-supplements/.

49. Challem, Jack, *"Licorice Twist"*. BetterNutrition. Web Retrieved May 1, 2016 from http://www.betternutrition.com/licorice-health-benefits/.

50. *"Diagnos-Techs" Test Panels.* Web Retrieved May 14, 2016 from http://www.diagnostechs.com/Pages/TestPanels.aspx.

51. Pepper M.D., Gary, *"What Are Bioflavonoids And Why Are They Helpful"*, (August 23, 2008). Metabolism.com. Web Retrieved May 17, 2016 from http://www.metabolism.com/2008/08/23/bioflavonoids-helpful/.

52. Jockers, Dr. David, "The superfood power of goji berries", (May 29, 2012). Natural News. Web Retrieved May 17, 2016 from http://www.naturalnews.com/036003_goji_berries_superf ood_nutrients.html.

53. Adams, Mike, *"Camu Camu: The Natural Vitamin C Powerhouse For Peak Mental Function and Nervous System Protection"*. Natural News. Web Retrieved May 17, 2016 from http://www.naturalnews.com/Report_Camu_Camu_1.html.

54. *"HEPA"*, Wikipedia.org. Web Retrieved August 7, 2016 from https://en.wikipedia.org/wiki/HEPA.

ABOUT THE AUTHOR

Thomas Calabris is a health and wellness coach. He has studied anatomy and physiology and many areas of natural health. He has studied and practiced many forms of meditation and Qigong for more than thirty years. He studied meditation, Qigong, and Tai Chi from Grandmaster Robert Krueger. He studied Inner Dan Arts Qigong (meditation, breathing, exercise, and healing) with Grandmaster Tianyou Hao. Thomas is a certified instructor of Inner Dan Arts Qigong. He also studied Qinway Qigong with Grandmaster Qinyin and Wisdom Healing Qigong with Master Mingtong Gu. He holds a Bachelor of Science Degree in Electrical Engineering and a Master of Science Degree in Biomedical Engineering. He is also a software engineer. He brings a unique perspective of science, tradition, and experience to his teachings. It is his mission to empower people to take charge of their health and wellness through natural and holistic practices like meditation, Qigong, Tai Chi, and healthy eating.

Learn more about stress relief at:
https://www.EliminateStressNow.com

Learn more about Qigong at:
http://www.InnerVitalityQigong.com

BOOKS BY THE AUTHOR

Relax Your Mind: Simple Meditation Techniques to Relieve Stress and Quiet a Busy Mind

Learn more at:
https://books2read.com/RelaxYourMind

Relax Your Mind Companion Workbook: A Guide to Learn Meditation Techniques to Relieve Stress and Quiet a Busy Mind

Learn more at:
https://books2read.com/RelaxYourMindWorkbook

The Color of Relaxation: Adult Coloring Book for Stress Relief and Relaxation

Learn more at:
https://www.eliminatestressnow.com/adultcoloringbookforstressrelief/

Dreams Into Reality: Manifest Your Dreams Into Being Using The Law of Attraction

Learn more at:
https://books2read.com/DreamsIntoReality

Healing Stress: Effective Solutions for Relieving Stress and Living a Stress-Free Life

Learn more at:
https://books2read.com/HealingStress

The Color of Mindfulness: Nature Mandalas Adult Coloring Book for Stress Relief and Relaxation

Learn more at:
https://www.eliminatestressnow.com/mindfuladultcoloringbookforstressrelief

Healthy Vegan Cooking: A Beginner's Guide To Plant-Based Cooking

Learn more at:
https://books2read.com/HealthyVeganCooking